Copyright ©

All rights reserved. No part of this publication may be reproduced, distributed, or transmitted in any form or by any means, including photocopying, recording, or other electronic or mechanical methods, without the prior written permission of the publisher, except in the case of brief quotations embodied in critical reviews and certain other noncommercial uses permitted by copyright law

Table of Contents

INTRODUCTION 4
CHAPTER ONE 6
    What Is Cancer 6
    Differences between Cancer Cells and Normal Cells 8
    How Cancer Arises 9
    Fundamentals of Cancer 11
    "Drivers" of Cancer 15
    When Cancer Spreads 17
Types of Cancer 19
    Carcinoma 20
    Sarcoma 22
    Leukemia 23
    Lymphoma 23
    Brain and Spinal Cord Tumors 25
CHAPTER TWO 28
    Acid Alkaline Basics 28
    what are acids and alkalines 29
    Balancing your pH 30
    Taking Charge of Your pH 32
    Making better choices 33
    Altering your diet 34
    Making Healthy Food Choices 34
    Getting Started 44

Top ten reasons to pay attention to your diet 44
CHAPTER THREE 47
Alkaline Diet for Cancer 47
What does "pH level" mean 53
How an Alkaline Diet Works 54
Alkaline Diet Benefits 56
How to Follow an Alkaline Diet 60
Best Alkaline Foods: 62
Alkaline Diet vs. Paleo Diet 66
Is the Alkali-rich Diet Good or Bad? 71
CONCLUSION 73

INTRODUCTION

The alkaline diet for cancer involves eating a special diet high in alkaline foods and low in acidic foods. This is suggested by advocates as a method of preventing cancer, slowing the growth of tumors and aiding in cancer treatments. Advocates believe that eating certain foods will alter the pH balance of the body, thus making the environment less hospitable to tumors, but these beliefs are not endorsed by the medical community.

Test tube studies have demonstrated a link between acidity and tumor growth. Tumors in test tubes grow more rapidly in acidic environment, and chemotherapy is more effective at killing tumors if the area around the tumor is more alkaline. However, doctors caution that this result will not necessarily translate to human beings, and that no human studies have demonstrated this connection. Furthermore, there is no evidence that an appropriately high level of alkaline pH could be achieved in the body as a result of the alkaline diet to have these effects, even if the link was proven in humans.

CHAPTER ONE

What Is Cancer

Cancer is the name given to a collection of related diseases. In all types of cancer, some of the body's cells begin to divide without stopping and spread into surrounding tissues.

Cancer can start almost anywhere in the human body, which is made up of trillions of cells. Normally, human cells grow and divide to form new cells as the body needs them. When cells grow old or become damaged, they die, and new cells take their place.

When cancer develops, however, this orderly process breaks down. As cells become more and more abnormal, old or damaged cells survive when they should die, and new cells form when they are not needed. These extra cells can divide without stopping and may form growths called tumors.

Many cancers form solid tumors, which are masses of tissue. Cancers of the blood, such as leukemias, generally do not form solid tumors.

Cancerous tumors are malignant, which means they can spread into, or invade, nearby tissues. In addition, as these tumors grow, some cancer cells can break off and travel to distant places in the body through the blood or the lymph system and form new tumors far from the original tumor.

Unlike malignant tumors, benign tumors do not spread into, or invade, nearby tissues. Benign tumors can sometimes be quite large, however. When removed, they usually don't grow back, whereas malignant tumors sometimes do. Unlike most benign tumors elsewhere in the body, benign brain tumors can be life threatening.

Differences between Cancer Cells and Normal Cells

Cancer cells differ from normal cells in many ways that allow them to grow out of control and become invasive. One important difference is that cancer cells are less specialized than normal cells. That is, whereas normal cells mature into very distinct cell types with specific functions, cancer cells do not. This is one reason that, unlike normal cells, cancer cells continue to divide without stopping.

In addition, cancer cells are able to ignore signals that normally tell cells to stop dividing or that begin a process known as programmed cell death, or apoptosis, which the body uses to get rid of unneeded cells.

Cancer cells may be able to influence the normal cells, molecules, and blood vessels that surround and feed a tumor—an area known as the microenvironment. For instance, cancer cells can induce nearby normal cells to form blood vessels that supply tumors with oxygen and nutrients, which they need to grow. These blood vessels also remove waste products from tumors.

Cancer cells are also often able to evade the immune system, a network of organs, tissues, and specialized cells that protects the body from infections and other conditions. Although the immune system normally removes damaged or abnormal cells from the body, some cancer cells are able to "hide" from the immune system.

Tumors can also use the immune system to stay alive and grow. For example, with the help of certain immune system cells that normally prevent a runaway immune response, cancer cells can actually keep the immune system from killing cancer cells.

How Cancer Arises

Cancer is a genetic disease that is, it is caused by changes to genes that control the way our cells function, especially how they grow and divide.

Genetic changes that cause cancer can be inherited from our parents. They can also arise during a person's lifetime as a result of errors that occur as cells divide or because of damage to DNA caused by certain environmental exposures. Cancer-causing environmental exposures include substances, such as the chemicals in tobacco smoke, and radiation, such as ultraviolet rays from the sun. (Our Cancer Causes and Prevention section has more information.)

Each person's cancer has a unique combination of genetic changes. As the cancer continues to grow, additional changes will occur. Even within the same tumor, different cells may have different genetic changes.

In general, cancer cells have more genetic changes, such as mutations in DNA, than normal cells. Some of these changes may have nothing to do with the cancer; they may be the result of the cancer, rather than its cause.

Fundamentals of Cancer

Cancer cells can break away from the original tumor and travel through the blood or lymph system to distant locations in the body, where they exit the vessels to form additional tumors. This is called metastasis.

Cancer is a disease caused when cells divide uncontrollably and spread into surrounding tissues.

Cancer is caused by changes to DNA. Most cancer-causing DNA changes occur in sections of DNA called genes. These changes are also called genetic changes.

A DNA change can cause genes involved in normal cell growth to become oncogenes. Unlike normal genes, oncogenes cannot be turned off, so they cause uncontrolled cell growth.

In normal cells, tumor suppressor genes prevent cancer by slowing or stopping cell growth. DNA changes that inactivate tumor suppressor genes can lead to uncontrolled cell growth and cancer.

Within a tumor, cancer cells are surrounded by a variety of immune cells, fibroblasts, molecules, and blood vessels—what's known as the tumor microenvironment. Cancer cells can change the microenvironment, which in turn can affect how cancer grows and spreads.

Immune system cells can detect and attack cancer cells. But some cancer cells can avoid detection or thwart an attack. Some cancer treatments can help the immune system better detect and kill cancer cells.

Each person's cancer has a unique combination of genetic changes. Specific genetic changes may make a person's cancer more or less likely to respond to certain treatments.

Genetic changes that cause cancer can be inherited or arise from certain environmental exposures. Genetic changes can also happen because of errors that occur as cells divide.

Most often, cancer-causing genetic changes accumulate slowly as a person ages, leading to a higher risk of cancer later in life.

Cancer cells can break away from the original tumor and travel through the blood or lymph system to distant locations in the body, where they exit the vessels to form additional tumors. This is called metastasis.

Cancer is a disease caused when cells divide uncontrollably and spread into surrounding tissues.

Cancer is caused by changes to DNA. Most cancer-causing DNA changes occur in sections of DNA called genes. These changes are also called genetic changes.

A DNA change can cause genes involved in normal cell growth to become oncogenes. Unlike normal genes, oncogenes cannot be turned off, so they cause uncontrolled cell growth.

In normal cells, tumor suppressor genes prevent cancer by slowing or stopping cell growth. DNA changes that inactivate tumor suppressor genes can lead to uncontrolled cell growth and cancer.

Within a tumor, cancer cells are surrounded by a variety of immune cells, fibroblasts, molecules, and blood vessels—what's known as the tumor microenvironment. Cancer cells can change the microenvironment, which in turn can affect how cancer grows and spreads.

Immune system cells can detect and attack cancer cells. But some cancer cells can avoid detection or thwart an attack. Some cancer treatments can help the immune system better detect and kill cancer cells.

Each person's cancer has a unique combination of genetic changes. Specific genetic changes may make a person's cancer more or less likely to respond to certain treatments.

Genetic changes that cause cancer can be inherited or arise from certain environmental exposures. Genetic changes can also happen because of errors that occur as cells divide.

Most often, cancer-causing genetic changes accumulate slowly as a person ages, leading to a higher risk of cancer later in life.

Cancer cells can break away from the original tumor and travel through the blood or lymph system to distant locations in the body, where they exit the vessels to form additional tumors. This is called metastasis.

"Drivers" of Cancer

The genetic changes that contribute to cancer tend to affect three main types of genes—proto-oncogenes, tumor suppressor genes, and DNA repair genes. These changes are sometimes called "drivers" of cancer.

Proto-oncogenes are involved in normal cell growth and division. However, when these genes are altered in certain ways or are more active than normal, they may become cancer-causing genes (or oncogenes), allowing cells to grow and survive when they should not.

Tumor suppressor genes are also involved in controlling cell growth and division. Cells with certain alterations in tumor suppressor genes may divide in an uncontrolled manner.

DNA repair genes are involved in fixing damaged DNA. Cells with mutations in these genes tend to develop additional mutations in other genes. Together, these mutations may cause the cells to become cancerous.

As scientists have learned more about the molecular changes that lead to cancer, they have found that certain mutations commonly occur in many types of cancer. Because of this, cancers are sometimes characterized by the types of genetic alterations that are believed to be driving them, not just by where they develop in the body and how the cancer cells look under the microscope.

When Cancer Spreads

ENLARGE

A cancer that has spread from the place where it first started to another place in the body is called metastatic cancer. The process by which cancer cells spread to other parts of the body is called metastasis.

Metastatic cancer has the same name and the same type of cancer cells as the original, or primary, cancer. For example, breast cancer that spreads to and forms a metastatic tumor in the lung is metastatic breast cancer, not lung cancer.

Under a microscope, metastatic cancer cells generally look the same as cells of the original cancer. Moreover, metastatic cancer cells and cells of the original cancer usually have some molecular features in common, such as the presence of specific chromosome changes.

Treatment may help prolong the lives of some people with metastatic cancer. In general, though, the primary goal of treatments for metastatic cancer is to control the growth of the cancer or to relieve symptoms caused by it. Metastatic tumors can cause severe damage to how the body functions, and most people who die of cancer die of metastatic disease.

Tissue Changes that Are Not Cancer

Not every change in the body's tissues is cancer. Some tissue changes may develop into cancer if they are not treated, however. Here are some examples of tissue changes that are not cancer but, in some cases, are monitored:

Hyperplasia occurs when cells within a tissue divide faster than normal and extra cells build up, or proliferate. However, the cells and the way the tissue is organized look normal under a microscope. Hyperplasia can be caused by several factors or conditions, including chronic irritation.

Dysplasia is a more serious condition than hyperplasia. In dysplasia, there is also a buildup of extra cells. But the cells look abnormal and there are changes in how the tissue is organized. In general, the more abnormal the cells and tissue look, the greater the chance that cancer will form.

Some types of dysplasia may need to be monitored or treated. An example of dysplasia is an abnormal mole (called a dysplastic nevus) that forms on the skin. A dysplastic nevus can turn into melanoma, although most do not.

An even more serious condition is carcinoma in situ. Although it is sometimes called cancer, carcinoma in situ is not cancer because the abnormal cells do not spread beyond the original tissue. That is, they do not invade nearby tissue the way that cancer cells do. But, because some carcinomas in situ may become cancer, they are usually treated.

Types of Cancer

There are more than 100 types of cancer. Types of cancer are usually named for the organs or tissues where the cancers form. For example, lung cancer starts in cells of the lung, and brain cancer starts in cells of the brain. Cancers also may be described by the type of cell that formed them, such as an epithelial cell or a squamous cell.

You can search NCI's website for information on specific types of cancer based on the cancer's location in the body or by using our A to Z List of Cancers. We also have collections of information on childhood cancers and cancers in adolescents and young adults.

Here are some categories of cancers that begin in specific types of cells:

Carcinoma

Carcinomas are the most common type of cancer. They are formed by epithelial cells, which are the cells that cover the inside and outside surfaces of the body. There are many types of epithelial cells, which often have a column-like shape when viewed under a microscope. Carcinomas that begin in different epithelial cell types have specific names:

Adenocarcinoma is a cancer that forms in epithelial cells that produce fluids or mucus. Tissues with this type of epithelial cell are sometimes called glandular tissues. Most cancers of the breast, colon, and prostate are adenocarcinomas.

Basal cell carcinoma is a cancer that begins in the lower or basal (base) layer of the epidermis, which is a person's outer layer of skin.

Squamous cell carcinoma is a cancer that forms in squamous cells, which are epithelial cells that lie just beneath the outer surface of the skin. Squamous cells also line many other organs, including the stomach, intestines, lungs, bladder, and kidneys. Squamous cells look flat, like fish scales, when viewed under a microscope. Squamous cell carcinomas are sometimes called epidermoid carcinomas.

Transitional cell carcinoma is a cancer that forms in a type of epithelial tissue called transitional epithelium, or urothelium. This tissue, which is made up of many layers of epithelial cells that can get bigger and smaller, is found in the linings of the bladder, ureters, and part of the kidneys (renal pelvis), and a few other organs. Some cancers of the bladder, ureters, and kidneys are transitional cell carcinomas.

Sarcoma

Sarcomas are cancers that form in bone and soft tissues, including muscle, fat, blood vessels, lymph vessels, and fibrous tissue (such as tendons and ligaments). Osteosarcoma is the most common cancer of bone. The most common types of soft tissue sarcoma are leiomyosarcoma, Kaposi sarcoma, malignant fibrous histiocytoma, liposarcoma, and dermatofibrosarcoma protuberans.

Leukemia

Cancers that begin in the blood-forming tissue of the bone marrow are called leukemias. These cancers do not form solid tumors. Instead, large numbers of abnormal white blood cells (leukemia cells and leukemic blast cells) build up in the blood and bone marrow, crowding out normal blood cells. The low level of normal blood cells can make it harder for the body to get oxygen to its tissues, control bleeding, or fight infections.

There are four common types of leukemia, which are grouped based on how quickly the disease gets worse (acute or chronic) and on the type of blood cell the cancer starts in (lymphoblastic or myeloid).

Lymphoma

Lymphoma is cancer that begins in lymphocytes (T cells or B cells). These are disease-fighting white blood cells that are part of the immune system. In lymphoma, abnormal lymphocytes build up in lymph nodes and lymph vessels, as well as in other organs of the body.

There are two main types of lymphoma:

Hodgkin lymphoma – People with this disease have abnormal lymphocytes that are called Reed-Sternberg cells. These cells usually form from B cells. Non-Hodgkin lymphoma – This is a large group of cancers that start in lymphocytes. The cancers can grow quickly or slowly and can form from B cells or T cells.

Multiple Myeloma

Multiple myeloma is cancer that begins in plasma cells, another type of immune cell. The abnormal plasma cells, called myeloma cells, build up in the bone marrow and form tumors in bones all through the body. Multiple myeloma is also called plasma cell myeloma and Kahler disease.

Melanoma

Melanoma is cancer that begins in cells that become melanocytes, which are specialized cells that make melanin (the pigment that gives skin its color). Most melanomas form on the skin, but melanomas can also form in other pigmented tissues, such as the eye.

Brain and Spinal Cord Tumors

There are different types of brain and spinal cord tumors. These tumors are named based on the type of cell in which they formed and where the tumor first formed in the central nervous system. For example, an astrocytic tumor begins in star-shaped brain cells called astrocytes, which help keep nerve cells healthy. Brain tumors can be benign (not cancer) or malignant (cancer).

Other Types of Tumors

Germ Cell Tumors

Germ cell tumors are a type of tumor that begins in the cells that give rise to sperm or eggs. These tumors can occur almost anywhere in the body and can be either benign or malignant.

Neuroendocrine Tumors

Neuroendocrine tumors form from cells that release hormones into the blood in response to a signal from the nervous system. These tumors, which may make higher-than-normal amounts of hormones, can cause many different symptoms. Neuroendocrine tumors may be benign or malignant.

Carcinoid Tumors

Carcinoid tumors are a type of neuroendocrine tumor. They are slow-growing tumors that are usually found in the gastrointestinal system (most often in the rectum and small intestine). Carcinoid tumors may spread to the liver or other sites in the body, and they may secrete substances such as serotonin or prostaglandins, causing carcinoid syndrome.

CHAPTER TWO

Acid Alkaline Basics

Alkaline-forming foods provide myriad health benefits. Focusing on elderly diets, the same study found that alkaline foods, including fresh vegetables, helped the elderly combat acids in dietary proteins and improve their ability to retain healthy muscle mass. Mom knew what she was talking about when she told you to eat your veggies!

Acid-forming foods are bad for you. But you may not realize the danger, because the damage starts inside, where you can't see it. Out of sight, out of mind — sadly, that's how many view their diet-health connection. They can't see the damage acid-forming foods are causing, so they don't do anything to change it.

On an acid alkaline diet you see the results of the foods you eat when you measure your pH. These measurements reflect the acid-alkaline balance in your body.

what are acids and alkalines

Everything in the universe has an opposing force night and day, yin and yang, and, of course, acid and alkaline. On a linear 0 to 14 pH scale, acidic substances (think stomach acid) range from the lowest pH of 0 to 7. Vinegar, for instance, has a pH reading of about 2.0 (acidic). Conversely, alkaline substances (think minerals) fall between 7 and 14 on the scale. Calcium, which is highly alkaline, has a pH around 10.

Every food (and drink) you ingest has the potential to form acid or alkaline ash during digestion. This leftover slush of chemicals has the potential to alter your body's pH environment, which is how foods are categorized as "acid forming" or "alkaline forming."

Balancing your pH

An acid alkaline diet doesn't require fancy supplements or prepackaged meals. The whole point is to help your body balance its pH, which is the overall measurement of acids and bases (also called alkalines) throughout your body. Your body is naturally alkaline (pH greater than 7.0) and functions at its best when it's more alkaline. However, chronically eating acid-forming foods (think red meat) tips your pH balance out of whack and sets the stage for illness.

Your pH balance influences every single function in your body, from breathing to digestion. You have the ability to influence your pH through diet and lifestyle by making more alkaline choices.

Ignoring the unenlightened

During your journey to pH balance, you may come across people colleagues, friends, even family members who either don't understand the acid alkaline diet or openly preach that it's a fraudulent fad. I implore you to keep this thought in the back of your mind at all times:

<mark>How can eating a diet composed largely of natural vegetables, fruits, and lean proteins not have excellent outcomes?</mark> Day-glow orange socks and jelly bracelets are fads; eating for your health is not.

We should know better by now

In the American northeast, nestled in the woods of Beltsville, Maryland, lies the Beltsville Human Nutrition Research Center. Their claim to fame is that they were the first facility to compile a research study detailing the effects of diet and nutrition in humans. According to their website, this occurred around the 1890s.

By the 20th century, even Samuel Clemens, more widely known as Mark Twain (1835-1910), knew about diet and health publications as evidenced by his famous quote,

"Be careful about reading health books. You may die of a misprint."

Now, in the 21st century, we have almost too much information at our fingertips, yet we continue to pollute our systems with unpronounceable chemicals, fatty foods, and acids.

==Today, everyone knows that dietary choices impact the human body in== myriad ways and that poor food choices lead to disease. Now is the time to start doing something about it.

Taking Charge of Your pH

Yes, you can control your pH balance, as well as how hard your body has to work to keep it in check. If you're constantly putting acids in your body, it's constantly working to remove said acids and doesn't have time for much else.

Acids in your body are like a poorly behaved five year old in the grocery store. He's running down the aisles tipping soda bottles over and dumping displays of food. Your body, (the store clerk) is constantly pulling a "clean up on Aisle 7" routine. With all that extra work, the clerk doesn't have time to restock shelves, place orders, or care for the general upkeep of the store. It's time to take charge of your pH and stop letting the five year old run amuck.

Making better choices

Working toward a healthy, balanced pH is as straightforward as choosing a carrot over a puffed orange crunchie. Although I demonstrate how to check urine pH measurements, keep logs, and even make shopping lists, you don't have to do any of that to enjoy the benefits of being more alkaline today than you were yesterday.

Your success on the acid alkaline diet boils down to choice you can fill three-quarters of your plate with fresh vegetables or with processed foods. The vegetables contain vitamins, fiber, and alkalinizing minerals, whereas the processed food contains acidifying chemicals, fatty acids, cholesterol, and probably excessive calories and sodium. Your choice.

Altering your diet

You will have to alter what you eat on the acid alkaline diet, but you won't have to go crazy and donate half the food in your fridge to local shelters. You don't have to pretend you can permanently abstain from your comfort foods that almost always leads to giving up on a diet.

Instead, there are ways to minimize these comfort foods while still enjoying them and make alkaline-forming foods the star on your plate..

Making Healthy Food Choices

Soon you'll understand how to differentiate when it's safe to tell your inner five year old "no" and when you can say "yes." He's going to sit on your shoulder and beg for a grilled cheese, a cold glass of milk, and a helping of French fries. You don't have to quit eating everything you enjoy, you just need to discover how to select more alkaline-forming foods and fill your plate with them.

What I'm encouraging you to eat

The purpose of eating more alkaline-forming foods is twofold:

✓ You decrease the amount of acid-forming foods you munch on, which allows your body to take a break from correcting your pH and focus on general housekeeping boosting your immune system, recovering from disease or illness, and so on.

✓ A consistently alkaline pH allows your body to start fixing acid build-up and all of the health problems associated with it, such as digestive disorders or skin problems. Now that you're no longer bombarding your body with acids, it can focus on healing itself and repairing damage. Alkaline-forming foods are synonymous with healthy foods and include:

✓ Vegetables

✓ Fruits (natural, not sweetened or dried)

✓ Sprouted grains

✓ Almonds and lentils

✓ Tofu and soy products

What to stop eating

You should limit the acid-forming foods to encompass between 20 and 40 percent of your plate, tops. Acid-forming foods come in shades of gray you have a choice of lean animal proteins (poultry), that are the least acid-forming, and you have the atomic bomb of acid proteins, which are your fatty red meats and wild game. Some examples of the acid-forming foods include:

• Red and processed meats

- Fried and fatty foods

- Whole dairy products

- Yeasty breads and wheat products

- Sugar-laden snacks and beverages.

Although these foods should be limited, you can enjoy the occasional sweet treat or fatty morsel.

Finding hidden acids

Take a walk to your pantry. Do you see ketchup, mayonnaise, salad dressings, croutons, and coffee? They're what I like to call the hidden acids, and each of them impacts your pH in a bad way. I could proclaim myself a health freak because I had a piece of toast for breakfast, salad for lunch and chicken breast for dinner. What I forgot to mention was the fact that my toast was smothered in jelly, my salad was awash in ranch-style dressing, and my chicken breast was fried all of a sudden it's not so healthy when you take off the rose-colored glasses.

These tiny, seemingly inconsequential hidden acids add up! Acid-forming foods are acid-forming foods no matter the size. Take a piece of broccoli and drench it in cheese sauce. You just nixed the alkaline-forming potential of that amazing vegetable. Don't render your alkaline-forming foods null and void; embrace their natural flavors, and leave the sauces, gravies, and condiments to someone else.

How Food and Life Impact pH

Your health is a long-term investment. I know it sounds really easy for me to sit here saying, "quit doing (insert bad habit here)." I realize that habits, such as tobacco use, poor dietary choices, or even a sedentary lifestyle, are very hard to break

The human body maintains a slightly alkaline pH, sometimes to your detriment. If acids are running amuck in your system, your body leeches calcium and other minerals from your bones to neutralize them. Rather than letting your acidic pH balance treat your bones like an ATM for calcium, it's better to cut out some of the acid-forming substances in your life.

Some lifestyle-acquired acids that can ruin your pH include:

✓ Smoking and tobacco use

✓ Drinking alcohol

✓ Leading a sedentary life

✓ Overdoing the workouts

✓ Ingesting coffee, soda, and other stimulants

✓ Using recreational drugs

✓ Being consistently dehydrated (not drinking enough water)

Reversing the Damage

The human body has an almost miraculous ability to heal, but only if you give it the right tools. Instead of rationalizing poor choices by saying the damage's already done, you can use that energy to power a lifestyle and dietary change aimed toward wellness.

For every ten men or women diagnosed with a dietary-impacted illness (diabetes, high blood pressure, and anemia, for example), I'd bet over half of them didn't change their lifestyle or diet after diagnosis. Many illnesses can be halted, if not reversed, through diet alone.

Taking baby steps

Change one thing in favor of your pH balance, or change absolutely everything it's up to you. But experts agree that taking small steps toward a goal is the best way to reach it.

Habits like Tracking calories, ounces, and macronutrients is required at every meal and snack.

Make lists of "good" foods and "bad" ones. It is not certain if the diet is useful.

It is not advised for anyone trying the diet to come too far out of their comfort zone. If the recipes with tofu freak you out, avoid them. If you faint at the site of vegetables, start by cutting some acid-forming foods out of your diet (red meats, sodas). Then, you can build on that small but sturdy foundation one step at a time.

Tracking changes

Tracking your pH measurements may help illustrate your results. You can't predict when you'll start seeing results from a balanced pH diet, nor could anyone. But if you put pen to paper and start tracking those daily morning pH results (as well as how you feel), you can see the changes for yourself.

' Embracing Health

Sometimes you simply make bad dietary choices on purpose. You know you should've avoided that jelly-filled donut, but you wanted it. Embracing health can be as easy as understanding that for every dietary choice you make, there's a reaction in your body good or bad. It's a little more complicated than eat grilled pickles and get diarrhea, but the concept's similar.

Some of the ways an acid alkaline balanced diet can help you improve your health include:

• Increased fiber in your diet leads to a healthier colon, decreased cholesterol, increased weight control, and manageable blood sugars.

• Decreased saturated fats promotes a healthier cardiovascular system (heart, arteries), easier weight control, and a decreased risk of stroke.

• Increased nutrients gives your body the right tools vitamins, minerals, and phytochemicals to function as it was meant to.

So there's no potion, pill, or device you need to enjoy an acid alkaline diet just healthy foods!

It's absolutely heartbreaking when it does occur, but, fortunately chronic diseases are not as common in children as they are in their adult counterparts. This is because they've not polluted their little bodies yet they're still functioning on all cylinders. The majority of people don't show symptoms of chronic illness (high blood pressure, fatigue, weight gain) until they're in their 40s. Fact.

Years of acid-forming foods, environmental pollution, and chemical invasion add up. Truth: Your cells have a natural life cycle, and every cell in your body will die at some point. Another truth: You can hasten said life cycle by chemically polluting your cells.

I wish I could tell you exactly what symptom to look for, but I can't. Years of chronic acidity manifest differently in each of us. You have an individual fingerprint; likewise, your individual genes, or DNA, dictate your weakest link. Mine is skin; an acid-eating party results in an acne outbreak. You may have a nervous system weakness, with lethargy and irritability your only outward symptoms of an imbalanced pH. Chances are, you already know where your systemic weakest link lies.

Getting Started

Before you get started, it is very important for anyone with an existing disease or condition who hopes to cure it through diet. First, congrats to you for taking charge of your body, nutrition, and lifestyle. However, Please talk to your doctor before you get started. Changes in diet can affect medical treatment and prescription regiments, and it is not good to lose the benefit of any treatment or drug.

Top ten reasons to pay attention to your diet

A poor diet, which means consistently eating unhealthy foods, can set the stage for disease in your body. It's like issuing an invitation to a hungry vampire — you open the door to disease and it's going to come in. Check out these diseases that may be preventable with attention to diet and nutrition:

- Anemia
- Certain cancers (such as colon, bladder, and breast)
- Colds and flu virus
- Diabetes
- Gallstones
- Gout
- Heart disease (includes high blood pressure, cholesterol, and heart attack)
- Metabolic syndrome (a collection of symptoms, such as high blood pressure and a large midsection, that may herald more serious diseases, such as diabetes)
- Obesity
- Stroke

Shut the door on disease (and vampires) by eating a healthy, balanced diet full of vitamins and minerals. Proven fact: You can cut your risk of many diseases with proper nutrition.

Staying the course

If excuses were worth money, I'd be a rich woman. It's human nature to rationalize bad decisions, so I'm not picking on anyone. I only encourage reflecting on why you stopped a healthy diet, exercise, or lifestyle. Was it too hard? Not fiscally feasible? No results?

The acid alkaline diet is a lifelong journey. You won't be done with it in a few months (hopefully). There are no complications in eating healthy, alkaline forming foods for the rest of your life.

Giving yourself time to adjust

You're going to want to quit at some point. You may rationalize that you already feel better, it's too hard, or you just plain want to stop and go back to a more comfortable, let alone unhealthy, way of eating.

Give your body some time to get accustomed to the alkaline-forming foods. Many of them, like the cruciferous veggies, are full of fiber and can cause bloating and gas until you get accustomed to the extra fiber. But trust me, your colon will dance a jig when it realizes that these healthy foods are here to stay and that you've stopped filling it with chemicals and processed foods.

CHAPTER THREE

Alkaline Diet for Cancer

Alkaline diet: What cancer patients should know

There's so much information surrounding cancer and diet that it can be hard to separate the myths from the facts. That's especially true when it comes to trendy diets.

The alkaline diet is one such trendy diet that often comes up in conversations about both cancer treatment and prevention.

So, to learn more about this diet we talked to Maria Petzel, a senior clinical dietitian at MD Anderson. Here's what she had to say.

The alkaline diet is based on the theory that eating certain foods can change the body's acid levels, also called the pH levels. Some believe that changing the body's pH levels can improve your health and help you lose weight or even prevent cancer.

But there's no way the foods you eat can alter the pH level of your blood. The body's pH is a very tightly regulated system. If you change your diet, you may see changes in the pH of your saliva or urine because these are waste products, but there's no way you could ever eat enough that it really impacts your blood.

While we can't comment on specific brands, most alkaline water is just like bottled water with different mineral content. Alkaline water also can't change the pH of your blood.

What is the link between the alkaline diet and cancer?

Some studies have shown that acidic environments help cancer cells grow. So the idea is that a diet high in alkaline foods (high pH) and low in acidic foods will raise the body's pH levels (make the body more alkaline) and prevent or even cure cancer.

It should be noted that these are studies of cancer cells in a dish and do not represent the complex nature of how tumors behave in the human body. And food cannot change the pH of your blood.

What should cancer patients know before changing their diets

Research shows that there's no one diet or food that can cure cancer. But proper nutrition can help you feel your best during cancer treatment – or at any time.

That's why it's so important to talk to a doctor or a dietitian before beginning a new diet. This is true regardless of whether you have cancer. Different diet plans work for different people, and your doctor or dietitian can help you determine if a new diet will help you reach your health goals.

Your dietitian can assess your nutrition and talk with you about your nutrition goals, which may change at different stages of treatment. Your dietitian can help limit your diet's adverse effects on your treatment, minimize side effects and help you cope with new food sensitives that you've developed since your diagnosis.

Together, you and your clinical dietitian can find the right diet to help you feel your best. There are all types of diets out there some good, some bad but there is perhaps no diet better for longevity and staving off disease than an alkaline diet. Don't just take my word for it.

A 2012 review published in the Journal of Environmental Health found that balancing your body's pH through an alkaline diet can be helpful in reducing morbidity and mortality from numerous chronic diseases and ailments — such as hypertension, diabetes, arthritis, vitamin D deficiency, and low bone density, just to name a few.

How do alkaline diets work? Research shows that diets consisting of highly alkaline foods — fresh vegetables, fruits and unprocessed plant-based sources of protein, for example — result in a more alkaline urine pH level, which helps protect healthy cells and balance essential mineral levels. This can be especially important for women intermittent fasting and/or on the keto diet, as hormone levels can be altered.

Alkaline diets (also known as the alkaline ash diets) have been shown to help prevent plaque formation in blood vessels, stop calcium from accumulating in urine, prevent kidney stones, build stronger bones, reduce muscle wasting or spasms, and much more.

An alkaline diet also known as the alkaline ash diet, alkaline acid diet, acid ash diet, acid alkaline diet and even sometimes the pH diet — is one that helps balance the blood pH level of the fluids in your body, including your blood and urine. Your pH is partially determined by the mineral density of the foods you eat. All living organisms and life forms on earth depend on maintaining appropriate pH levels, and it's often said that disease and disorder cannot take root in a body that has a balanced pH.

The principles of the acid ash hypothesis help make up the tenets of the alkaline diet. According to research published in Journal of Bone and Mineral Research, "The acid-ash hypothesis posits that protein and grain foods, with a low potassium intake, produce a diet acid load, net acid excretion (NAE), increased urine calcium, and release of calcium from the skeleton, leading to osteoporosis." The alkaline diet aims to prevent this from happening by carefully taking food pH levels into consideration in an attempt to limit dietary acid intake.

Although some experts might not totally agree with this statement, nearly all agree that human life requires a very tightly controlled pH level of the blood of about 7.365–7.4. As Forbe's Magazine puts it, "Our bodies go to extraordinary lengths to maintain safe pH levels." Your pH can range between 7.35 to 7.45 depending on the time of day, your diet, what you last ate and when you last went to the bathroom. If you develop electrolyte imbalances and frequently consume too many acidic foods — aka acid ash foods — your body's changing pH level can result in increased "acidosis."

What does "pH level" mean

What we call pH is short for the potential of hydrogen. It's a measure of the acidity or alkalinity of our body's fluids and tissues. It's measured on a scale from 0 to 14. The more acidic a solution is, the lower its pH. The more alkaline, the higher the number is. A pH of around 7 is considered neutral, but since the optimal human body tends to be around 7.4, we consider the healthiest pH to be one that's slightly alkaline, and pH levels vary throughout the body, with the stomach being the most acidic region.

Even very tiny alterations in the pH level of various organisms can cause major problems. For example, due to environmental concerns, such as increasing CO_2 deposition, the pH of the ocean has dropped from 8.2 to 8.1 and various life forms living in the ocean have greatly suffered. The pH level is also crucial for growing plants, and therefore it greatly affects the mineral content of the foods we eat. Minerals in the ocean, soil and human body are used as buffers to maintain optimal pH levels, so when acidity rises, minerals fall.

How an Alkaline Diet Works

Here's some background on acid/alkalinity in the human diet, plus key points about how alkaline diets can be beneficial:

- Researchers believe that when it comes to the total acid load of the human diet, "there have been considerable changes from hunter gather civilizations to the present." Following the agricultural revolution and then mass industrialization of our food supply over the last 200 years, the food we eat has significantly less potassium, magnesium and chloride, along with more sodium, compared to diets of the past.

- Normally, the kidneys maintain our electrolyte levels (those of calcium, magnesium, potassium and sodium). When we're exposed to overly acidic substances, these electrolytes are used to combat acidity.

- According to the Journal of Environmental Health review mentioned earlier, the ratio of potassium to sodium in most people's diets has changed dramatically. Potassium used to outnumber sodium by 10:1, however now the ratio has dropped to 1:3. People eating a "Standard American Diet" now consume three times as much sodium as potassium on average!

- Many children and adults today consume a high-sodium diet that's very low in not only magnesium and potassium, but also antioxidants, fiber and essential vitamins. On top of that, the typical Western diet is high in refined fats, simple sugars, sodium and chloride.

- All of these changes to the human diet have resulted in increased "metabolic acidosis." In other words, the pH levels of many people's bodies are no longer optimal. On top of this, many are suffering from low nutrient intake and problems such as potassium and magnesium deficiency.

- This accelerates the aging process, causes gradual loss of organ functions, and degenerates tissue and bone mass. High degrees of acidity force our bodies to rob minerals from the bones, cells, organs and tissues.

Alkaline Diet Benefits

1. Protects Bone Density and Muscle Mass

Your intake of minerals plays an important role in the development and maintenance of bone structures. (5) Research shows that the more alkalizing fruits and vegetables someone eats, the better protection that person might have from experiencing decreased bone strength and muscle wasting as they age, known as sarcopenia.

An alkaline diet can help balance ratios of minerals that are important for building bones and maintaining lean muscle mass, including calcium, magnesium and phosphate. Alkaline diets also help improve production of growth hormones and vitamin D absorption, which further protects bones in addition to mitigating many other chronic diseases.

2. Lowers Risk for Hypertension and Stroke

One of the anti-aging effects of an alkaline diet is that it decreases inflammation and causes an increase in growth hormone production. This has been shown to improve cardiovascular health and offer protection against common problems like high cholesterol, hypertension (high blood pressure), kidney stones, stroke and even memory loss.

3. Lowers Chronic Pain and Inflammation

Studies have found a connection between an alkaline diet and reduced levels of chronic pain. Chronic acidosis has been found to contribute to chronic back pain, headaches, muscle spasms, menstrual symptoms, inflammation and joint pain.

One study conducted by the Society for Minerals and Trace Elements in Germany found that when patients with chronic back pain were given an alkaline supplement daily for four weeks, 76 of 82 patients reported significant decreases in pain as measured by the "Arhus low back pain rating scale." (6)

4. Boosts Vitamin Absorption and Prevents Magnesium Deficiency

An increase in magnesium is required for the function of hundreds of enzyme systems and bodily processes.

Many people are deficient in magnesium and as a result experience heart complications, muscle pains, headaches, sleep troubles and anxiety. Available magnesium is also required to activate vitamin D and prevent vitamin D deficiency, which is important for overall immune and endocrine functioning.

5. Helps Improve Immune Function and Cancer Protection

When cells lack enough minerals to properly dispose of waste or oxygenate the body fully, the whole body suffers. Vitamin absorption is compromised by mineral loss, while toxins and pathogens accumulate in the body and weaken the immune system.

Research published in the British Journal of Radiologyshowed that cancerous cell death (apoptosis) was more likely to occur in an alkaline body. (7) Cancer prevention is believed to be associated with an alkaline shift in pH due to an alteration in electric charges and the release of basic components of proteins. Alkalinity can help decrease inflammation and the risk for diseases like cancer — plus an alkaline diet has been shown to be more beneficial for some chemotherapeutic agents that require a higher pH to work appropriately.

6. Can Help You Maintain a Healthy Weight

Limiting consumption of acid-forming foods and eating more alkaline-forming foods can protect your body from obesity by decreasing leptin levels and inflammation, which affects your hunger and fat-burning abilities. Since alkaline-forming foods are anti-inflammatory foods, consuming an alkaline diet gives your body a chance to achieve normal leptin levels and feel satisfied from eating the amount of calories you really need.

How to Follow an Alkaline Diet

Here are some key tips for following an alkaline diet:

Whenever possible, try to buy organic alkaline foods. Experts feel that one important consideration in regard to eating an alkaline diet is to become knowledgeable about what type of soil your produce was grown in — since fruits and vegetables that are grown in organic, mineral-dense soil tend to be more alkalizing. Research shows that the type of soil that plants are grown in can significantly influence their vitamin and mineral content, which means not all "alkaline foods" are created equally.

The ideal pH of soil for the best overall availability of essential nutrients in plants is between 6 and 7. Acidic soils below a pH of 6 may have reduced calcium and magnesium, and soil above a pH of 7 may result in chemically unavailable iron, manganese, copper and zinc. Soil that's well-rotated, organically sustained and exposed to wildlife/grazing cattle tends to be the healthiest.

If you're curious to know your pH level before implementing the tips below, you can test your pH by purchasing strips at your local health food store or pharmacy. You can measure your pH with saliva or urine. Your second urination of the morning will give you the best results. You compare the colors on your test strip to a chart that comes with your test strip kit. During the day, the best time to test your pH is one hour before a meal and two hours after a meal. If you test with your saliva, you want to try to stay between 6.8 and 7.2.

Best Alkaline Foods:

• Fresh fruits and vegetables promote alkalinity the most. Some of the top picks include mushrooms, citrus, dates, raisins, spinach, grapefruit, tomatoes, avocado, summer black radish, alfalfa grass, barley grass, cucumber, kale, jicama, wheat grass, broccoli, oregano, garlic, ginger, green beans, endive, cabbage, celery, red beet, watermelon, figs and ripe bananas.

• All raw foods: Ideally try to consume a good portion of your produce raw. Uncooked fruits and vegetables are said to be biogenic or "life-giving." Cooking foods depletes alkalizing minerals. Increase your intake of raw foods, and try juicing or lightly steaming fruits and vegetables.

• Plant proteins: Almonds, navy beans, lima beans and most other beans are good choices.

• Alkaline water: Alkaline water has a pH of 9 to 11. Distilled water is just fine to drink. Water filtered with a reverse osmosis filter is slightly acidic, but it's still a far better option than tap water or purified bottled water. Adding pH drops, lemon or lime, or baking soda to your water can also boosts its alkalinity.

• Green drinks: Drinks made from green vegetables and grasses in powder form are loaded with alkaline-forming foods and chlorophyll. Chlorophyllis structurally similar to our own blood and helps alkalize the blood.

• Other foods to eat on an alkaline diet include sprouts, wheatgrass, kamut, fermented soy like natto or tempeh, and seeds.

Anti-Alkaline Foods and Habits:

Foods that contribute most to acidity include:

- High-sodium foods: Processed foods contain tons of sodium chloride — table salt — which constricts blood vessels and creates acidity.

- Cold cuts and conventional meats

- Processed cereals (such as corn flakes)

- Eggs

- Caffeinated drinks and alcohol

- Oats and whole wheat products: All grains, whole or not, create acidity in the body. Americans ingest most of their plant food quota in the form of processed corn or wheat.

- Milk: Calcium-rich dairy products cause some of the highest rates of osteoporosis. That's because they create acidity in the body! When your bloodstream becomes too acidic, it will steal calcium (a more alkaline substance) from the bones to try to balance out the pH level. So the best way to prevent osteoporosis is to eat lots of alkaline green leafy veggies!

- Peanuts and walnuts

- Pasta, rice, bread and packaged grain products

What other kinds of habits can cause acidity in your body? The biggest offenders include:

- Alcohol and drug use

- High caffeine intake

- Antibiotic overuse

- Artificial sweeteners

- Chronic stress

- Declining nutrient levels in foods due to industrial farming

- Low levels of fiber in the diet

- Lack of exercise

- Excess animal meats in the diet (from non-grass-fed sources)

- Excess hormones from foods, health and beauty products, and plastics

- Exposure to chemicals and radiation from household cleansers, building materials, computers, cell phones and microwaves

- Food coloring and preservatives

- Over-exercise

- Pesticides and herbicides

- Pollution

- Poor chewing and eating habits

- Processed and refined foods

- Shallow breathing

Alkaline Diet vs. Paleo Diet

- The Paleo diet and alkaline diet have many things in common and a lot of the same benefits, such as lowered risk for nutrient deficiencies, reduced inflammation levels, better digestion, weight loss or management, and so on.

- Some things that the two have in common include eliminating added sugars, reducing intake of pro-inflammatory omega-6 fatty acids, eliminating grains and processed carbs, decreasing or eliminating dairy/milk intake, and increasing intake of fruits and veggies.

- However, there are several important things to consider if you plan to follow the Paleo diet. The Paleo diet eliminates all dairy products, including yogurt and kefir, which can be valuable sources of probiotics and minerals for many people — plus the Paleo diet doesn't always emphasize eating organic foods or grass-fed/free-range meat (and in moderation/limited quantities).

- Additionally, the Paleo diet tends to include lots of meat, pork and shellfish, which have their own drawbacks.

- Eating too many animal sources of protein in general can actually contribute to acidity, not alkalinity. Beef, chicken, cold cuts, shellfish and pork can contribute to sulfuric acid buildup in the blood as amino acids are broken down. Try to obtain the best quality animal products you can, and vary your intake of protein foods to balance your pH level best.

Alkaline Diet for Cancer

First, let us understand what a high-alkali diet plan is. This is a diet which includes foods that have high alkali and low acid content. A high-alkali foods list would include items such as squash, lettuce, tomatoes, celery, carrots, onions, spinach, cucumber, chickpeas, parsley, basil, olive oil, limes and lemons, watermelons, etc. On the other hand, food items like meat, eggs, pasta, sugar, caffeine, tobacco, white rice, etc., have high acid content. Studies have proved that certain types of cancer cells flourish well in an acidic environment, whereas, high alkali content in the blood stunts their growth and spread. Laboratory experiments have even proved that chemotherapy shows better cancer fighting results if the area surrounding the cancer has an alkaline environment.

However, the counter argument refuting the claims of alkali-rich diet benefits with regards to cancer state that, while it has been proved in test-tube environment that alkalies are effective in killing cancer cells, it has not been proved in any actual human study. Also, refuters of this diet (which include many noted oncologists and medical practitioners) claim that the body has several mechanisms through which it automatically restores the pH balance, preventing increase or decrease of both acid and alkali content. Therefore, deliberately increasing alkali content of the body by switching to a high alkali diet won't have any effect for any significant length of time, thereby, ruling out the possibility of having sufficient time to interact with cancer cells.

How Does it Work

Cancer cells are anaerobic which means that they cannot survive in an oxygen rich environment. Most of us are aware that the more hydrogen content a compound has the more acidic it is whereas the more oxygen molecules a compound has, the more alkaline it tends to be. Therefore, when the blood and tissues are oxygen rich, it means that all the toxins are eliminated which ensures that cancerous tissues do not thrive in such environment. Alkali rich tissues are capable of holding 20 times more oxygen than acidic tissues, thereby further ruling out the growth of cancer cells. When the acid content in the blood increases, it usually deposits the extra acid in some tissue of the body to rid itself and restore the pH balance. This deposited acid eventually kills some of the surrounding cells which, again, turn acidic. Metabolic disorders like acid reflux, constipation, etc., are most common causes of increased blood acid content. Doctors often recommend alkaline foods for acid reflux and constipation treatment.

Is the Alkali-rich Diet Good or Bad?

A completely alkali-oriented diet may eventually backfire as complete exclusion of acids means that you totally abolish certain food groups that actually help you fight cancer. For instance, a totally alkaline diet rules out inclusion of dairy products which are a major source of vitamin D. The fact that sufficient intake of vitamin D boosts a person's cancer survival capacity has been clinically proven. Therefore, although it is true that cancer flourishes in an acidic environment and acid rich foods encourage the growth and spread of cancer, a completely alkaline diet is not recommended either. Often, a high-alkali diet for weight loss is recommended to people who do not benefit from low carb or fad diets. A combined diet of a higher percentage of alkaline and lower ratio of acidic food is good for those who suffer from stress and chronic acidity. Extremity in anything is harmful. Therefore, maintaining moderation is a must when tampering with the body's pH balance.

As we can see, the concept of alkaline diet to counter cancer is a disputed concept. While on one hand, scientific proof surrounding properties of acids, alkali, and cancerous cells point towards the capability of an alkali-rich diet to curb cancer, the lack of human evidence and the body's tendency to balance all excesses (whether of acids or alkali) etch a serious question mark upon this much debated, controversial topic.

CONCLUSION

While these findings are accurate, they apply only to cells in an isolated lab setting. Altering the cell environment of the human body to create a less-acidic, less-cancer-friendly environment is virtually impossible.

While proponents of this myth argue that avoiding certain foods and eating others can change the body's pH level, these claims stand in stark contrast to everything research shows about the chemistry of the human body.Acid-base balance is tightly regulated by several mechanisms, among them kidney and respiratory functions. Even slight changes to your body's pH are life-threatening events. Patients with kidney disease and pulmonary dysfunction, for example, often rely on dialysis machines and mechanical ventilators (respectively) to avoid even small disruption of acid-base balance.

Home "test kits," which measure the pH of urine, do not relay information about the body's pH level. Foods, drinks and supplements will affect the acidity or alkalinity of urine, but it is the only fluid that is affected. In fact, excess acid or base is excreted in the urine to help maintain proper pH balance in the body.

Made in the USA
Las Vegas, NV
01 May 2021

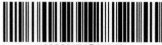